YOUR KNOWLEDGE HAS VALUE

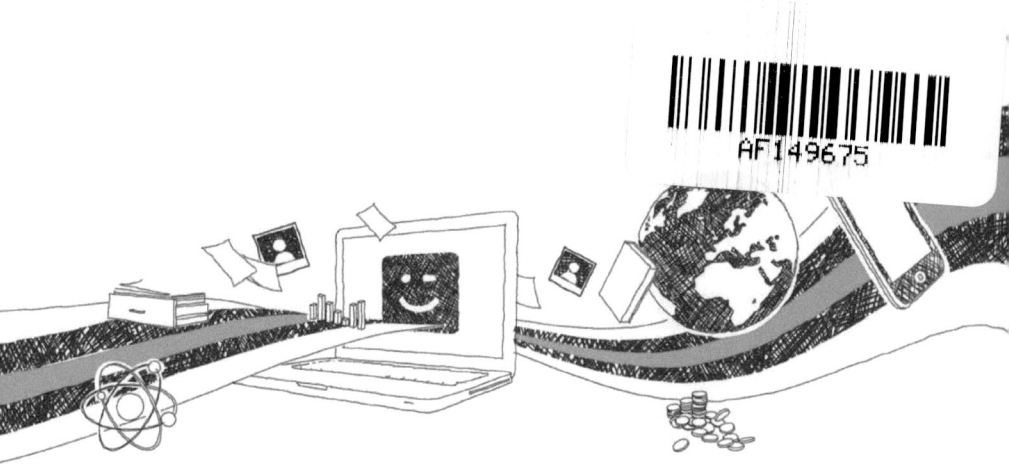

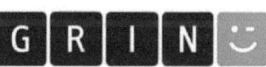

Mark Zaidi

Scientific Literature Review: X-linked Adrenoleukodystrophy

GRIN Publishing

Bibliographic information published by the German National Library:

The German National Library lists this publication in the National Bibliography; detailed bibliographic data are available on the Internet at http://dnb.dnb.de .

Imprint:

Copyright © 2014 GRIN Verlag GmbH
Print and binding: Books on Demand GmbH, Norderstedt Germany
ISBN: 978-3-656-86726-5

This book at GRIN:

http://www.grin.com/en/e-book/285279/scientific-literature-review-x-linked-adrenoleukodystrophy

GRIN - Your knowledge has value

Since its foundation in 1998, GRIN has specialized in publishing academic texts by students, college teachers and other academics as e-book and printed book. The website www.grin.com is an ideal platform for presenting term papers, final papers, scientific essays, dissertations and specialist books.

Visit us on the internet:

http://www.grin.com/

http://www.facebook.com/grincom

http://www.twitter.com/grin_com

Scientific Literature Review:

X-linked Adrenoleukodystrophy

Full Name: **Mark Zaidi**

Date Submitted: **12/03/2014**

Introduction

In 1984, there was a young boy named Lorenzo Odone. He was a gifted

child who was fluent in not only English, but French and Italian as well.

Unfortunately, shortly after his 6th birthday, he experienced several unusual

symptoms, such as speech problems, worsening hand-eye coordination, and

decreased hearing. His mother recalls the day during which she was reading him a

story, and as he snuggled up to her, Lorenzo complained that he could not hear

well. Shortly after that, Lorenzo was diagnosed with X-linked

Adrenoleukodystrophy (X-ALD).

X-ALD is a rare and irreversible disease, which progressively degrades the

brain and nervous system. Doctors had given him 2 years left to live. However, his

father, Augusto, was not ready to give up. Regardless of having no prior medical

knowledge, Augusto devoted his life to finding a cure for X-ALD. Even though he

was unable to cure Lorenzo (and X-ALD for that matter), he managed to prolong

his life for two decades, thanks to a medicine he invented, named "Lorenzo's oil",

in memory of his son. This story is an example of how one man's love for his son

sparked scientific research in the treatment of a debilitating disorder. Even though

there is no strong scientific proof that Lorenzo's oil helps decrease the effects of

X-ALD, it undoubtedly increased the quality of Lorenzo's life.

Topic Statement

This scientific literature review will address X-ALD through case studies that demonstrate the clinical features of the disorder. It will also discuss the genetic, metabolic and biochemical aspects, and treatment options of X-ALD, and areas of future research.

Case Study

In this section, we will explore several case studies, as well as the symptoms of X-ALD. The first two case studies reviewed here are those of a seven-year-old male child (Case 1) and a six-year-old male child (Case 2).

Case 1 presented primarily with decreased hearing. The child seemed to have had relatively normal motor dexterity in all four limbs but abnormal tendon reflexes. Magnetic Resonance Imaging (MRI) produced the following image (Figure 1) (Rai, 2013). In this image, abnormal brain signal activity has been noted in the cerebral white matter, in forms of patchy and/or bilaterally symmetrical spots. This description is similar to that of X-ALD patients.

Case 2 presented with more severe symptoms. The child was born to a non-consanguineous couple (parents were not related). He had delayed developmental milestones, compared to that of an average child. Additionally, he presented with approximately five instances of non-projectile vomiting in a period of six months.

Hyperpigmentation was evident in his oral cavities, skin, and nails. Similarly to

Case 1, he had relatively normal motor dexterity in all four limbs, but had

abnormal tendon reflexes. The MRI of Case 2 (Figure 2) was similar to that of

Case 1. It showed abnormalities in the cerebral white matter, in forms of patchy

and/or bilaterally symmetrical spots (Rai, 2013). Additionally, another key

symptom depicted by Case 2 was the abnormally high level of Very Long Chain

Fatty Acids (VLCFAs), which were observed on his blood test results (Figure 3)

(Rai, 2013).

     Our last case study is that of a 37-year-old Korean man (Case 3) (Kang,

2014). Unlike the other two cases, he had bladder incontinence, difficulty

speaking, and motor-dexterity problems. Additionally, Case 3 is different from the

other two cases in that the symptoms arose much later in the patient's life.

Additional research showed a *de novo* mutation (a mutation that was not inherited

from his parents) located on exon 1 at nucleotide position c.277_296dup20

(p.Ala100Cysfs*10) of the adenosine *triphosphate-binding cassette D1* (*ABCD1*)

gene (Kang, 2014). The MRI of Case 3 (Figure 4) was very similar to that of the

other two cases, however the brainstem seemed to be relatively unaffected (Kang,

2014).

     To summarize the clinical aspects of X-ALD, this disorder does not have

one set of symptoms, but rather a unique set for each of its phenotypes. If diagnosed from 3 to 10 years of age, it will classify as the "childhood cerebral form", which is the progressive degeneration of neurons and white matter, resulting in a comatose state if left untreated. The "adolescent form" is from 11-21 years of age, and has a less severe phenotype than that of the "childhood cerebral form". "Adrenomyeloneuropathy" (AMN) occurs in patients aged 21-37 years, and results in progressive neuropathy and paraparesis. The "adult cerebral form" is from 38 years onwards, and results in dementia and behavioural abnormalities. However, one must note that these are not perfectly discrete forms of the disorder, as symptoms can differ from case to case. For example in Case 2, the non-projectile vomiting was not an expected symptom.

Genetics

In this section, we will be discussing the location of the gene responsible for X-ALD on the chromosome, as well as its function. X-ALD is caused by a mutation in the ATP-binding *cassette sub-family D member 1 (ABCD1)* gene ("Genetics Home Reference", 2014). X-ALD is an X-linked variant of ALD, meaning that the affected gene causing the disorder is located on the X chromosome. The normal function of this gene is to produce the Adrenoleukodystrophy Protein (ALDP). The purpose of this protein is to bring VLCFAs in through the peroxisome membrane, in order for the peroxisomes to break them up. However, due to a mutation, ALDP is unable to bind to the

VLCFAs, therefore they cannot be brought into the peroxisomes and begin to accumulate in the body. Due to this accumulation, they damage the nervous system in ways that will be further discussed in the "Biochemical Aspects" section.

X-ALD is considered a relatively rare disorder, as its estimated occurrence is anywhere between 1 : 20 000 to 1 : 100 000 males worldwide (Moser, 1997). There is no seeming predominance for any race, as patients have been identified from many races and geographic locations, such as Americans, Chinese, and Africans. *ABCD1* is located on the long (q) branch at position 28 of the X chromosome (Xq28) ("Genetics Home Reference", 2014). More precisely, the *ABCD1* gene is located from base pair 153,724,867 to base pair 153,744,761 on the X chromosome (Figure 5) ("Genetics Home Reference", 2014).

Biochemical Aspects

In this section, we will explore the biochemical aspects of X-ALD, and contrast the function of the normal ABCD1 protein with its malfunctioning version. As mentioned earlier, X-ALD is caused by a mutation in the *ABCD1* gene, resulting in malformation of ALDP. Normally, ALDP is membrane-bound and sits on the peroxisome's membrane. VLCFAs binds to the protein and are carried inside the peroxisome to be broken down into hydrogen peroxide (Figure 6)

(Braverman, 2012). However, due to the mutation, the protein is unable to bind to the VLCFAs and as a result they start to build up.

Excess VLCFAs have many adverse effects. For example, they are toxic to the adrenal glands and could lead to adrenal gland failure. They wear away the myelin sheath (protective layer) of neurons (white matter), and can limit the functionality of neurotransmitters. Research suggests that the accumulation of VLCFAs triggers an inflammatory response in the brain, which could lead to the breakdown of myelin, also known as demyelination ("Genetics Home Reference", 2014). The damaging of these tissues leads to the previously discussed symptoms of X-ALD, such as dementia, motor problems and hearing loss.

Continuing Research

In this final section, we will discuss the continuing research on X-ALD, as well as current and newly developed methods of symptom treatment, such as Lorenzo's Oil, intrathecal baclofen, *ABCD2* overexpression, and allogeneic hematopoietic stem cell transplantation. Unfortunately, X-ALD is currently an incurable disease that ultimately leads to death. However, there has been some recent research on multiple ways to manage the symptoms, and therefore increase the lifespan of a patient suffering with the disease. One of the most famed treatments is that of a mixture of triglycerides known as "Lorenzo's Oil".

Lorenzo's Oil is a mixture of 4 parts glyceryl trioleate and 1 part glyceryl

trierucate (Moser, 1997). While there is no hard scientific evidence that Lorenzo's

Oil is a reliable treatment option, there have been multiple cases in which patients

treated with the supplement exceeded their predicted life expectancy by over 10

years, such as in Lorenzo Odone's case. His story provoked notable interest from

the film industry, to the point where it became a major motion picture in 1992.

This was perhaps one of the most influential times for X-ALD awareness. Prior to

the film, the general public knew little about the disorder since it is relatively rare.

Another, more recent possible treatment, is the utilization of intrathecal

baclofen. Baclofen's original use was to treat spastic disorders such as multiple

sclerosis and cerebral palsy, because it is a chemical that facilitates muscle

relaxation. However, scientists have successfully used a pump to maintain a

continuous infusion of Baclofen into the spinal cord of an 8-year-old X-ALD

patient. This significantly decreased the amount and severity of spasms that the

patient experienced, and restored a little bit of voluntary muscle movement (Chu,

2001).

Another hypothetical treatment option is the overexpression of the *ABCD2*

gene to compensate for the mutated *ABCD1* (Weber, 2014). *ABCD2* is a close

homologue to *ABCD1*, having a 63% amino acid similarity ("Genetics Home

Reference", 2014). Through pharmacological means, the artificial overexpression of *ABCD2* produces the Adrenoleukodystrophy Related Protein (ALDRP), which can be used to perform ALDP's function, bringing VLCFAs into the peroxisome.

Finally, there is allogeneic hematopoietic stem cell transplantation as a potential treatment for X-ALD. This is the process of taking the healthy stem cells from the umbilical cord of a recently conceived healthy sibling, and transplanting them into the patient with X-ALD (Moser, 1997). This process would effectively halt the demyelination process, but must be done at an early age to be effective. Additionally, it requires the conception of a healthy child shortly after the affected one is born, in order to attain umbilical cord stem cells that are genetically a good match for the affected patient (Moser, 1997).

Conclusion

X-ALD is a devastating and incurable disease, in which the accumulation of VLCFAs results in the demyelination and inflammation of cerebral white matter. This ultimately leads to the key symptoms of X-ALD, such as dementia, hearing impairment and loss of motor abilities. The accumulation of VLCFAs is due to a mutation in the *ABCD1* gene, which results in a malfunctioning protein that is unable to carry VLCFAs into the peroxisome for degradation. X-ALD is an X-linked disease, as the mutated *ABCD1* gene is located at Xq28. Even though there is no cure for X-ALD, there are numerous viable treatment options, such as Lorenzo's Oil, intrathecal baclofen, *ABCD2* overexpression, and allogeneic hematopoietic stem cell transplantation, all of which aim to prolong survival and improve the quality of life of patients with X-ALD. More research is certainly needed to produce novel therapeutic approaches in the hopes of finding a cure for X-ALD in the future.

Figures

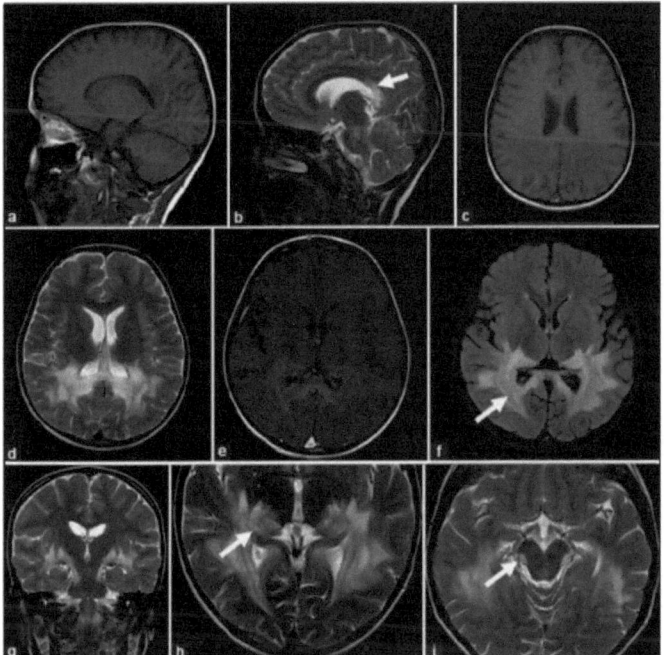

Figure 1: MRI of Case 1 showing abnormal signal intensities in the cerebral white matter (highlighted by the arrows) (Rai, 2013).

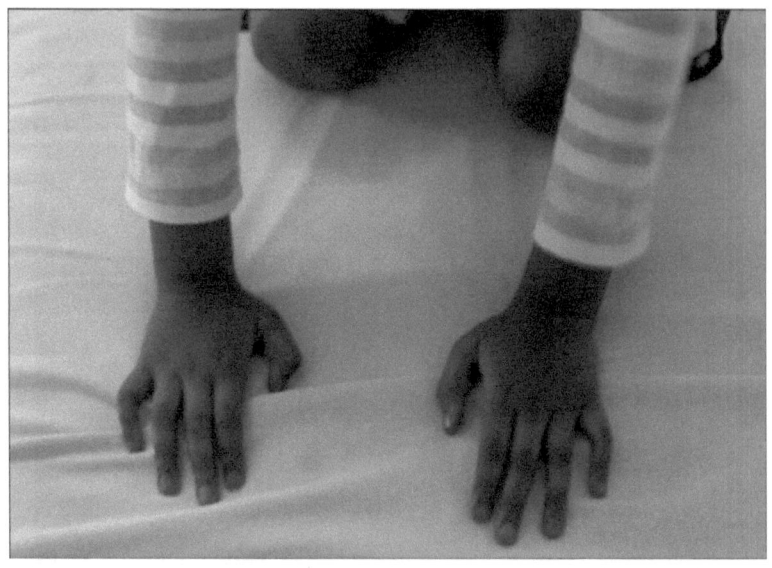

Figure 2: Hyperpigmentation of the skin and nails in Case 2 (Rai, 2013).

Test	Flag	Results	Unit	Reference Value	Perform Site*
Fatty Acid Profile, Comprehensive, S			REPORTED 12/02/2011 13:52		
Octanoic Acid, C8:0		13	nmol/mL	9-41	MCR
Decenoic Acid, C10:1		3.7	nmol/mL	1.6-6.6	MCR
Decanoic Acid, C10:0		6	nmol/mL	3-25	MCR
Lauroleic Acid, C12:1		3.8	nmol/mL	1.3-5.8	MCR
Lauric Acid, C12:0		61	nmol/mL	5-80	MCR
Tetradecadienoic Acid, C14:2		1.9	nmol/mL	0.2-5.8	MCR
Myristoleic Acid, C14:1		17	nmol/mL	1-31	MCR
Myristic Acid, C14:0		168	nmol/mL	40-290	MCR
Hexadecadienoic Acid, C16:2		19	nmol/mL	3-29	MCR
Hexadecenoic Acid, C16:1w9		45	nmol/mL	24-82	MCR
Palmitoleic Acid, C16:1w7		174	nmol/mL	100-670	MCR
Palmitic Acid, C16:0		1514	nmol/mL	960-3460	MCR
g-Linolenic Acid, C18:3w6		53	nmol/mL	9-130	MCR
a-Linolenic Acid, C18:3w3		37	nmol/mL	20-120	MCR
Linoleic Acid, C18:2w6	H	3932	nmol/mL	1600-3500	MCR
Oleic Acid, C18:1w9		1467	nmol/mL	350-3500	MCR
Vaccenic Acid, C18:1w7	L	193	nmol/mL	320-900	MCR
Stearic Acid, C18:0		772	nmol/mL	280-1170	MCR
EPA, C20:5w3	H	323	nmol/mL	6-90	MCR
Arachidonic Acid, C20:4w6	H	1040	nmol/mL	350-1030	MCR
Mead Acid, C20:3w9		16	nmol/mL	7-30	MCR
h-g-Linolenic Acid, C20:3w6		116	nmol/mL	60-220	MCR
Arachidic Acid, C20:0		54	nmol/mL	30-90	MCR
DHA, C22:6w3	H	852	nmol/mL	30-160	MCR
DPA, C22:5w6		23	nmol/mL	10-50	MCR
DPA, C22:5w3		153	nmol/mL	30-270	MCR
DTA, C22:4w6		11	nmol/mL	10-40	MCR
Docosenoic Acid, C22:1		4	nmol/mL	4-13	MCR
Docosanoic Acid, C22:0		46.4	nmol/mL	0.0-96.3	MCR
Nervonic Acid, C24:1w9		84	nmol/mL	50-130	MCR
Tetracosanoic Acid, C24:0		77.6	nmol/mL	0.0-91.4	MCR
Hexacosenoic Acid, C26:1	H	1.5	nmol/mL	0.3-0.7	MCR
Hexacosanoic Acid, C26:0	H	5.14	nmol/mL	0.00-1.30	MCR
Pristanic Acid, C15:0(CH3)4		0.10	nmol/mL	0.00-2.98	MCR
Phytanic Acid, C16:0(CH3)4		1.01	nmol/mL	0.00-9.88	MCR
Triene Tetraene Ratio		0.015		0.013-0.050	MCR
Total Saturated		2.7	mmol/L	1.4-4.9	MCR
Total Monounsaturated		2.0	mmol/L	0.5-4.4	MCR
Total Polyunsaturated	H	6.6	mmol/L	1.7-5.3	MCR

Figure 3: Table showing concentrations of VLCFAs in the blood plasma of Case 2. The abnormally high values are shown in boxes (Rai, 2013).

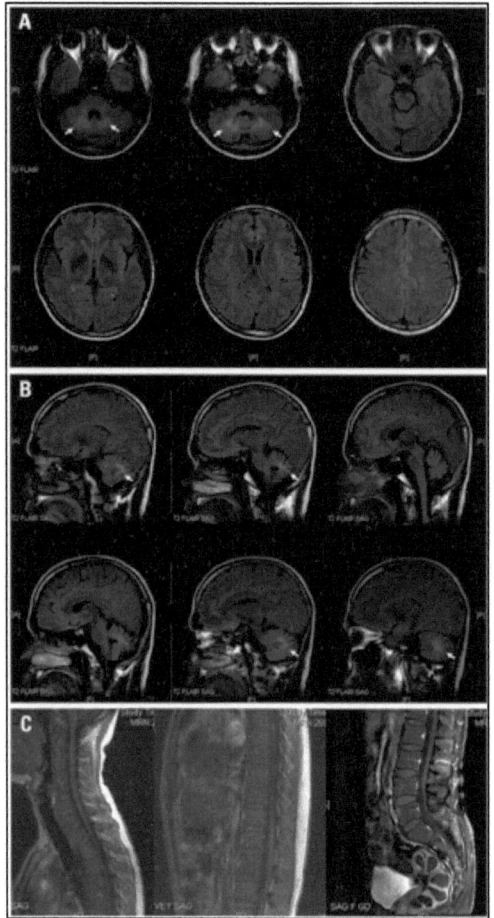

Figure 4: (A) MRI showing degradation of the denate nuclei and cerebral white matter (white arrows). **(B)** Fluid-attenuated inversion recovery MRI of the brain showed hyperintense lesions in the dentate nuclei (white arrows). **(C)** No contrast change was noted with gadolinium injection. (Kang, 2014)

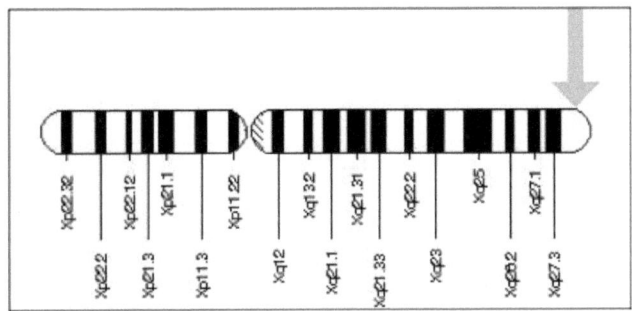

Figure 5: Image showing location of ABCD1 on the X chromosome. ("Genetics Home Reference", 2014)

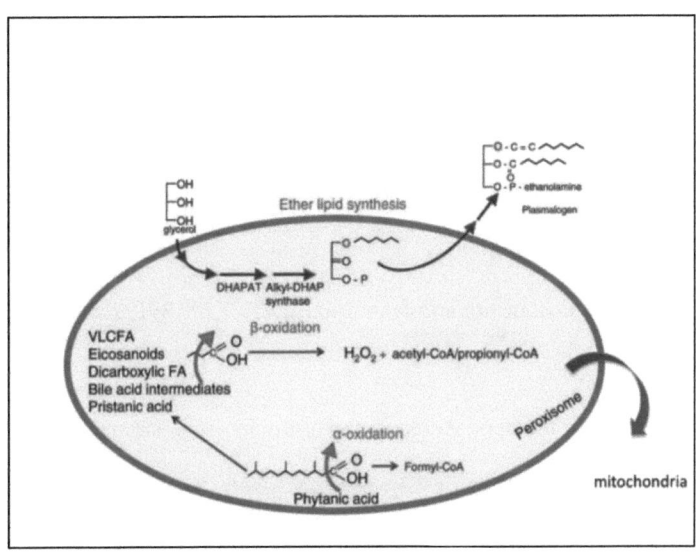

Figure 6: Diagram showing the regular process of VLCFAs degradation. The malfunctioning ABCD1 protein is unable to bring VLCFAs into the peroxisome, resulting in an accumulation outside of the peroxisome.

References

1. Moser, H. Adrenoleukodystrophy: Phenotype, Genetics, Pathogenesis and Therapy. 1997. *Brain.* 120(8):1485-1508. Retrieved October 9, 2014, from http://brain.oxfordjournals.org/content/brain/120/8/1485.full.pdf

2. Kang, J. et al. Isolated Cerebellar Variant of Adrenoleukodystrophy with a de novo Adenosine Triphosphate-Binding Cassette D1 (ABCD1) Gene Mutation. 2014. *Yonsei Med J.* 55(4):1157-1160. Retrieved October 8, 2014, from http://www.eymj.org/DOIx.php?id=10.3349/ymj.2014.55.4.1157

3. Weber, F. et al. Evaluation of Retinoids for Induction of the Redundant Gene ABCD2 as an Alternative Treatment Option in X-Linked Adrenoleukodystrophy. 2014. PLoS One. 9(7):e103742. Retrieved October 9, 2014, from http://www.plosone.org/article/info%3Adoi%2F10.1371%2Fjournal.pone.01 03742

4. Rai, S. et al. Childhood Adrenoleukodystrophy – Classic and Variant – Review of Clinical Manifestations and Magnetic Resonance Imaging. 2013. J Pediatr Neurosci. 8(3):192-197. Retrieved October 9, 2014, from http://www.ncbi.nlm.nih.gov/pmc/articles/PMC3888033/

5. Chu, M. et al. Intrathecal Baclofen in X-linked Adrenoleukodystrophy. 2001. Pediatr Neurol. 24(2): 156-158. Retrieved October 9, 2014, from http://www.pedneur.com/article/S0887-8994(00)00250-2/fulltext

6. Genetics Home Reference (2014/11/24). X-linked adrenoleukodystrophy. Retrieved November 25, 2014 from http://ghr.nlm.nih.gov/condition/x-linked-adrenoleukodystrophy

7. Braverman, N. (2012/6/26). Challenges to Therapy for X-linked Adrenoleukodystrophy. Retrieved November 29, 2014 from http://www.slideserve.com/hija/challenges-to-therapy-for-x-linked-adrenoleukodystrophy